AT
OFFICE
YOGA

Your At Work Yoga Guide
For Stiff Bodies That Sit All Day

By: Julie Schoen and Little Pearl

Love Yoga?
Check Out The Rest of The Just Do Yoga Series!

GOOD DAY YOGA
GOOD NIGHT YOGA
HAPPY BACK YOGA
FLAT TUMMY YOGA
STRESS LESS YOGA
SUPER IMMUNITY YOGA

Disclaimers
This book contains general information and is for informational purposes only. You should use proper discretion, and consult with a health care practitioner, before following any of the exercises, techniques, or plans described in this book. The author and publisher expressly disclaim responsibility for any adverse effects that may result from the use or application of the information contained in this book.

CONTENTS:

**1. Danger Zone: The Harmful Effects of
Your Office Chair and How Yoga Can Help**   **1**

2. Incorporating Yoga Before, During, and After Work   **5**

    Pre-Work Yoga Session   5
    At-Work Yoga Session   18
    Post-Work Yoga Session   29

**3. Overtime: Your Top 10 At-Work Yoga
Questions Answered**   **40**

    What are the most effective stretches for preventing and
        relieving carpal tunnel syndrome?   40
    I have no choice but to sit at a desk all day – what should I do?   44
    I've heard about companies offering yoga classes during lunch
        or after work, how do I convince my boss?   45
    Not only does my body ache at my desk, but I am stressed out too!
        What are the best ways to alleviate stress while working?   46
    Do I have to bring a yoga mat and change to do yoga at work?   47
    Will people think I'm weird if I start doing yoga at my desk?   47
    How often should I take a break and stretch or do some yoga?   48
    Why does sitting all day make me so tired?   48
    Instead of sitting all day I stand all day. Are there any special
        yoga poses that can help me?   49
    Work gives me a headache! Can yoga help?   54

DANGER ZONE
The Harmful Effects of Your Office Chair And How Yoga Can Help

There are very few of us who have the luxury of not being trapped behind a desk for several hours every day. Even when work does not require us to be sitting in a chair, hands on the keyboard, we modern humans tend to choose to do so as a form of relaxation. But have you ever noticed how your body looks and feels when you are sitting or typing? It's not pretty and in reality it's anything but relaxing.

The chair itself is a modern invention, the solution to our evolving lifestyle, earning a spot in the forefront of our lives as we moved from active hunters, gatherers, and farmers to corporate 9 to 5-ers. And while it serves its purpose (in fact the idea of life without chairs seems oddly laughable), the chair is wreaking havoc on our bodies.

As you sit, your body shifts out of alignment – shoulders hunch, low back collapses, and hips tense as the muscles in the legs shorten and contract. The more you sit, the more accustomed your body gets to what it feels like when it is misaligned. Sitting starts to feel natural when really it is anything but! Take a moment to think about little kids; they have a very hard time sitting still. Why? It's uncomfortable for the human body! Any first grade teacher knows that if they don't give their young students frequent breaks there's trouble in store. The same should be true for adults as well, but it isn't because we have adapted – adapted to being uncomfortable and unhappy.

And it goes further than just being uncomfortable. A sedentary lifestyle makes your bottom literally expand (and by expand I mean get huge) from sitting for hours on end, day after day. More seriously than just outward appearance, long stretches of sitting put you at higher risk for disease and illness (like obesity, heart disease, and diabetes) and early death as well. As you sit, your body starts to shut down metabolically, which means fewer calories are burnt, circulation slows, and the chances of feeling depressed, lethargic, and moody skyrocket.

For this reason, many office mice soon turn into gym rats, hoping to balance out the hours of sitting with an hour or two of intense activity. Although the logic is there, the evidence is not. You simply can't undo the negative effects of too much sitting by working out before or after. Even if you are the fittest, most in shape person you know, but you sit for hours on end, you are still more likely to die earlier than a person who is not in as good of shape but who moves more frequently throughout the day.

In order to be healthy, feel good, and look awesome you have to start incorporating movement into your day – and a lot of it. It doesn't have to be hard and you don't even have to leave your desk. In a recent study of thermogenesis by researchers at the Mayo Clinic it was discovered that even just small movements, simple stretches, even tapping your feet, can mean the difference between being obese and staying healthy because even the smallest motions keep your body functioning and your metabolism running.

The answer to great health is smaller than you probably imagined and so easy there is absolutely no excuse why you can't get started now! You don't even have to stop working if you don't want to – just move! Guaranteed your body will feel so much better, your mind will clear, stress will dissipate, and you will start to feel like that little first grader again – excited about life and ready to take on anything!

Now who's with me?

INCORPORATING YOGA BEFORE, DURING, AND AFTER WORK

Even the simplest stretching routines added to your day can do wonders for your body by boosting metabolism, burning calories, reducing pain, and overall improving your quality of life. The more you move, the better! And the best part about yoga is that it doesn't just get you moving, but it is proven to help mitigate the harmful effects of stress as well!

If you can do just one of the following yoga sessions each day you will start to feel the difference in your mind and body almost immediately. But why stop there? Three brief yoga sessions each day will make you the happiest (and might I add best looking) worker bee at your office! Today is the day you start changing how you feel, look, and work – let's do this!

PRE-WORK YOGA SESSION

Perform this short yoga sequence each morning before work to help loosen the muscles of the hips and shoulders and also lengthen the spine before a long day of sitting.

1. Shoulder Opener with Strap

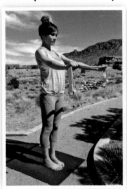 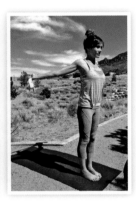

Stand tall with a strap (or dog leash, scarf, etc.) between your hands. It may take a few times to figure out exactly how far apart your hands should be, but a good place to start is a little wider than shoulder width. Straighten your arms out in front of you and as you inhale begin to lift the strap up and over your head. As you exhale, continue moving the strap behind you, keeping the arms straight and the chin lifted parallel to the ground. Inhale and bring the strap back up, exhaling as the strap returns to your starting position.

Your hands should be far enough apart that your arms can stay straight while moving through the entire range of motion, but close enough together that there is a slight degree of discomfort. As you feel these spots of discomfort (usually they happen as you move the strap behind you – there tends to be 3 "sticking" points) hold the strap there and breathe; the muscles should start to burn and tingle. If you rush through these tough areas you will be missing out on the healing benefits for the muscles of your shoulders and upper back. This exercise also is fantastic for creating incredible posture.

Perform this exercise 10 times at least, making sure you are not holding your breath or allowing the shoulders to hunch and the chin to move towards the chest.

2. **Marjaryasana and Bitilasana (Cat and Cow)**

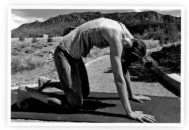

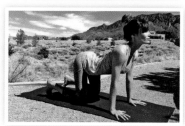

Come to all fours with hands under your shoulders and knees under your hips. Spread your fingers wide and press into the mat to help support your wrists. Start in Cat by rounding your spine and drawing the navel in towards the spine and up under the ribcage as you exhale. Allow your chin to tuck in towards your chest. Feel the stretch that you get in the upper back between the shoulders and the space that is created between each of your vertebrae. As you inhale, move forward into Cow by pressing your navel down towards the mat; open and broaden the chest while lifting your gaze.

Flow between these two postures several times (6 to 8 at the minimum) staying in tune with your breath. Do not rush the transition between the two postures; enjoy the opening and subtle movement of the spine with each tiny motion.

3. **Parivrtta Anjaneyasana (Revolved Low Lunge) – Insert Revolved Low Lunge**

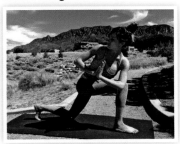

From all fours step your right foot forward so that the thigh becomes parallel to the ground and your ankle is directly under your knee. Bring your hands together at heart center and place the left elbow outside of the right thigh. Lengthen the spine by drawing the crown of the head forward and then deepen the twist by pressing the elbow against the thigh more.

To create stability and integrity in this posture, imagine pulling the heel of the right foot towards the back of your mat. Notice how this engages your front leg as well as prevents you from sinking down in the hips.

Hold this posture for 5 full breaths before coming back to all fours and repeating on the other side.

4. **Uttanasana (Standing Forward Bend),** *variation*

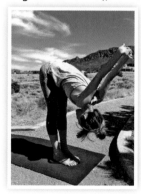

From Revolved Low Lunge, inhale and step the back foot forward to meet the front. Bring your toes together but keep the heels slightly apart. Clasp your hands behind your back and try to straighten your arms as you fold forward from your hips, straightening the legs as much as possible. Allow the head to be heavy so that your neck can relax and lengthen. Keep the legs strong and engaged by pulling the kneecaps up and rotating the upper inner thighs back. To more effectively perform this pose, pull the lower abdomen up and in. The spine should feel like it is lengthening while you are simultaneously opening the shoulders.

5. **Revolved High Lunge – Insert Revolved High Lunge**

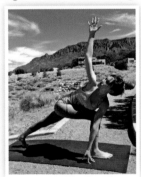

Release your hands from behind your back and return to stand in Tadasana (Mountain Pose). Step the left foot back and come into a high lunge. The back leg is straight with the heel off of the ground; press into the ball of the foot to help you balance. Make sure that your right knee tracks right over the ankle with the thigh parallel to the ground. Bring your left hand down to the ground on the inside of the foot. Reach the right arm up into the air, making one straight line with both arms. Lengthen the spine by reaching the crown of your head forward while continuing to anchor yourself with your back foot. Bring your gaze up to the top hand.

Hold this pose for 5 full breaths.

6. **Ardha Ustrasana (Half Camel Pose) – Insert Half Camel**

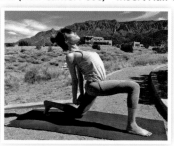

Drop your left knee to the mat from Revolved High Lunge. Clasp your hands behind your back and begin to run them down the back of your left leg. As you do this, lift the chest up towards the sky and squeeze the shoulder blades together. Because this pose is asymmetrical balance can be tough. Make sure you press firmly through all four corners of both feet in order to continue holding this pose as you move the hands further down your left leg.

Once you have reached the peak of your pose, hold for three breaths. When you exit the pose, make sure you come up slowly, head and chin last. If you feel dizzy or lightheaded at all, take a moment to rest in Balasana (Child's Pose) before continuing with your sequence.

7. Runner's Lunge

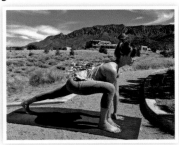

From Half Camel bring your hands to the front of your mat while walking your right foot over to the very edge of the mat. Lift the left knee off of the ground and keep the leg as straight as possible. Press through the heel of the back foot to intensify the stretch in the hip.

If this pose feels intense, stay here and hold for 5 breaths. If you feel like you can move into a deeper stretch, advance to the next pose.

8. **Utthan Pristhasana (Lizard Pose)**

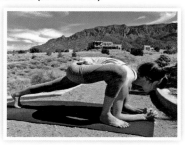

From Runner's Lunge, lower down onto your forearms. Do your best to keep the weight evenly distributed throughout the body, paying close attention to the balance between both arms. As you stretch the hip, notice if other areas of your body start to tense like the neck and face. Use the breath to help keep you relaxed and focused. Hold for 5 breaths.

Step forward to the top of the mat and take a breath in Tadasana (Mountain Pose). Return to Pose 4, Uttanasana, and repeat the poses on the other side.

9. Ustrasana (Camel Pose)

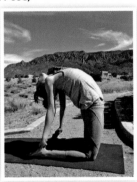

From Runner's Lunge or Lizard Pose, come to kneel at the top of your mat. Use two fists to measure the correct distance between your knees and then ensure that the knees and feet are lining up directly behind the knees as well. Bring your hands to your lower back and squeeze the elbows together as much as possible. Press the hips forward, working to get the knees, thighs, and hips in one line. As you do this, start to bend backwards and lift the chest up towards the sky, gently dropping the head and bending one vertebra at a time.

If you can go deeper into the pose, move your hands to your heels, keep pressing the hips forward and lifting the chest up. Because this pose is such an intense heart opener, know that you may feel intense emotions. Do your best to stay in this pose for 5 full breaths, using your breath to stay focused.

As you exit the pose move slowly, using your hands to support you on your way up, head and chin come up last.

10. **Balasana (Child's Pose),** *variation*

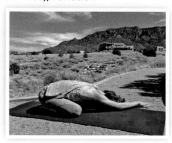

Immediately after Ustrasana, come into Balasana to release the intense back bend. Bring the toes together and the knees slightly apart. Fold over your thighs allowing your forehead to rest on the mat. Gently extend your arms with palms face down and elbows slightly bent in front of your body. Take a few breaths to rest in this position.

Walk your hands over to the right several inches and stack the left hand on top of the right. You should feel a nice opening in the left side body. Take 2 to 3 breaths on this side before walking your hands to the left and stretching the right side body.

11. Sasangasana (Rabbit Pose)

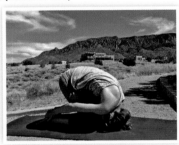

From Balasana (Child's Pose) return to all fours and bring the ankles and the sides of the feet together; sit back on your heels. Reach your hands back and get a firm grip on your heels, thumbs on the outside of the feet and the rest of your fingers on the inside. It's very important that you have a good grip so take some time to set yourself up here before entering the posture.

Holding onto the heels, begin to bring the crown of your head to the mat, forehead against the knees. If the forehead separates from the knees when the head comes down, walk your knees forward until they touch. Begin to pull on your heels and round the spine, lifting the hips up towards the sky, but not losing the grip whatsoever.

In this posture, approximately 15% of the weight should be on your head. If you feel like you have too much weight in the crown of your head, carefully come out of the posture the same way you entered and adjust your grip so that you are holding lower on the heel. The harder you pull on your heels the more compression you will create and the better benefits for your spine. Again, this is why grip is so important – pulling on the heels in this pose and losing the grip can cause you to fall forward and injure the neck and/or spine. Please perform this pose with caution and only try it once you have a thorough understanding.

Once in Rabbit, hold the position for 5 to 6 breaths, working to get deeper and deeper (more compressed) with each breath. As you are ready to exit the pose, come up slowly and with control, head and chin coming up last.

12. **Savasana (Corpse Pose),** *variation*

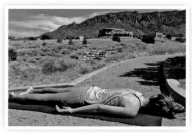

Unlike traditional Savasana, which is taken face up, try doing this pose lying on your stomach instead. Allow the toes to touch and heels to fall apart. Arrange the arms next to your body so that the palms face up and the elbows bend slightly. Place one ear on the mat while relaxing the muscles of the neck and face. Do your best to stay completely still in this posture, both physically and mentally. Let go of all tension in the body and feel the muscles start to loosen their grip on the bones. Still the mind by focusing on your breath, eventually allow the thought of your breath to completely dissipate as well. Rest here in Savasana for at least 2 minutes, longer if you have the time.

AT-WORK YOGA SESSION

The poses in this sequence can be done sequentially or it can be broken down and used throughout the day. All of these poses can be done seated (some require a chair), but remember that if you have the opportunity to do these stretches while standing take full advantage!

1. **Shoulder Circles**

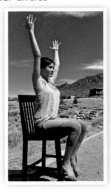 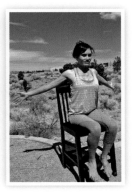

Sit up as tall as possible, lifting the chin so that it is parallel with the floor. Extend the arms out in front of you and begin to make slow circles with your arms, bringing the hands behind you, over your head, and then back in front. Do this several times in both directions, staying aware of your breathing and doing your best to connect the breath to the movements.

If space does not allow you to extend your arms fully, the same exercise can be done with the hands on the shoulders.

2. **Marjaryasana and Bitilasana (Cat and Cow),** *variation*

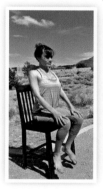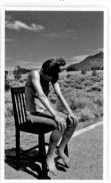

Sitting tall in the chair, bring your hands to your thighs. As you inhale, lift the chest towards the ceiling and squeeze the shoulder blades together. Lift the chin and bring your gaze up. As you exhale, round the upper back and bring the chin into the chest. Pull the navel towards the spine and under the ribcage. Enjoy the stretching of the upper back and neck. Do at least 5 cycles.

3. **Uttanasana (Forward Bend),** *variation*

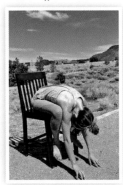

Sitting in your chair, spread your legs several inches apart and plant the feet firmly on the ground. Hinging forward from the hips, allow your body to rest between your legs. The arms and shoulders should dangle completely loose with the hands resting on the floor or wherever they can comfortably reach. Feel the spine and neck lengthen and relax. Avoid any gripping of the jaw or face. Take 5 to 6 full breaths before slowly rolling back up to sit one vertebra at a time.

4. Neck Stretch

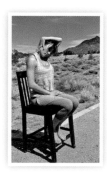

Sitting tall, reach your left arm straight up into the air. Reach the left hand over your head and place it on the outside of the right jaw. Squeeze your head in between your hand and bicep so that the weight of the head is completely supported and the neck relaxes. Using the left hand, begin to press the head towards the left shoulder. To intensify the stretch, start to lower the chin down towards the chest until you feel a good stretch all through the right side of the neck and into the upper back.

Hold this stretch for several breaths before repeating on the other side.

5. Bikram Ardha Chandrasana (Bikram Half Moon), *variation*

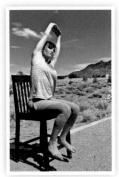

Sit tall in your chair and interlace the fingers above your head, palms facing the ceiling. Lift the chest up, keeping the chin parallel with the floor. Reach the arms as high above your head as possible. Then begin to bend to the right. Continue pressing through the palms of your hands, keeping the chest open by moving the left shoulder back slightly and the right shoulder forward.

Hold this stretch for 3 to 5 breaths before returning to center, switching the grip of your fingers, and repeating on the left side.

6. **Ustrasana (Camel Pose),** *variation*

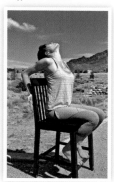

Reach your arms behind the chair. Depending on the style of the chair you will either interlace your fingers behind the back or hook the elbows over the top of the chair and press the palms of the hands into the back of it. Squeeze the shoulder blades together to help open the chest. Lift the chest towards the ceiling as much as possible, dropping the head back slightly.

Hold this pose for 4 to 5 breaths.

7. Ardha Garudasana (Half Eagle Pose)

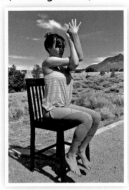

Reach your arms straight out in front of you, palms facing each other. Cross the right arm over the left at the elbows. Bring the right wrist under the left and the palms of the hands together in prayer position. Lift the elbows up until the backs of the arms are parallel with the floor. Start to press the forearms forward, trying to get them perpendicular to the floor. Breathe into the joints of arms and the upper back. Be sure to keep the shoulders and face relaxed.

Hold this position for 5 to 6 breaths and then repeat on the other side.

8. Seated Twist

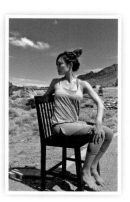

Sit up as tall as possible in your chair with your feet flat on the ground. Bring your left hand to the outside of the right thigh and your right hand to the back of your chair. As you inhale sit up taller. As you exhale twist deeper. The majority of the twist should be felt in the upper and mid back. If you are mainly feeling the stretch in your low back, make sure that your feet are firmly grounded and that your two knees are staying in one line. Hold this twist for 5 breaths and then repeat on the other side.

9. Seated Thread The Needle Fold

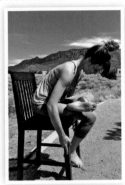

Sitting tall, bring the ankle of the left leg to the right thigh. Flex the left foot to help keep the knee safe. If this position feels intense, continue sitting as tall as possible, breathing into the hip and gluteus muscles to help them relax.

If your body is giving you space in this position, you can start to hinge forward from the hips to intensify the stretch. Hold this stretch for 8 to 10 breaths before repeating on the other side.

10. Uttana Shishosana (Extended Puppy Pose), *variation*

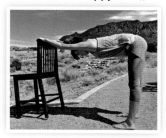

Stand behind your chair and grab onto the back of it. Walk as far away as necessary so that your arms can extend straight with your body making a 90-degree angle. Press your upper body down between your arms, keeping the back of the neck loose and legs straight. Hold this stretch for 8 to 10 breaths and repeat as many times as possible throughout the day!

11. **Viparita Karani (Legs-Up-The-Wall Pose),** *variation*

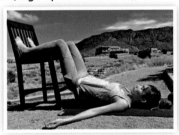

Come to sit on the floor facing your chair. Swing your legs up onto the seat of the chair and lie down flat on your back. Ideally your legs will create a 90-degree angle, but depending on the height of the chair this may or may not be possible. If your chair is higher than normal, try placing a block or pillow under your low back to help support you so that the legs can comfortably rest on the chair. If your chair is lower than usual, you might consider taking the feet to the back of the chair.

Once you have adjusted your pose so that you can comfortably rest, extend the arms out to your sides with palms facing up and elbows slightly bent. This pose is incredibly rejuvenating for the entire body and mind, but is especially beneficial for fatigued legs since you allow the blood that has collected in the feet and ankles to drain and replenish.

Stay in this pose for as long as you can (or until you get caught!)

POST-WORK YOGA SESSION

After a long day at work, yoga is the perfect solution to unwind, de-stress, and work out any of the kinks that may have collected in your body during the day.

1. **Balasana (Child's Pose),** *variation*

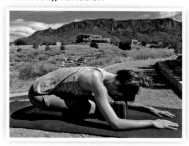

Kneeling in the center of your mat, spread the knees wide enough so that you can place a block between them. Lower your body down between your legs until the forehead touches the block. Keep the tops of the feet touching the ground and the hips close or in contact with your heels. Allow your hands to rest in front of you, palms down. Keep a slight bend in the elbows so that the shoulders can relax. Feel your breath move through your body and relax as you exhale out all of the worries and stresses of the day. Stay in this pose for 5 to 6 breaths, enjoying the complete relaxation that it provides.

2. **Wrist Stretch**

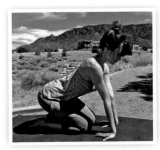

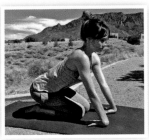

Kneeling in the center of your mat, place your hands in front of you, fingers pointing towards your knees. Press through the heel of the hand to help release tension in the wrists and fingers. Hold this position for 5 breaths.

Then, flip your hands over so that the palms of your hands face up. Press through the wrists until you feel a good stretch. Hold this position for 5 breaths.

3. Forearm Massage

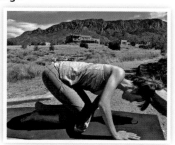

Place the forearm of your left arm on the mat, hand palm up. Using one or both of your knees begin to massage your forearm, wrist, and even the palm of the hand. You can adjust how much weight you apply to the arm to intensify this beneficial posture. Repeat with the other arm.

4. **Lazy Adho Mukha Svanasana
(Lazy Downward Facing Dog Pose)**

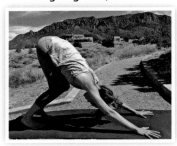

Come onto all fours and press back into Downward Facing Dog, keeping the knees bent. Your hands should be shoulder width apart and your feet hip width apart. Spread the fingers wide on the mat, lining up the index fingers with the long edges of your mat.

With the knees bent you can really focus on opening the shoulders and stretching the spine. To help spread the upper back, roll the upper inner arms back slightly. Relax the back of the neck so that the ears move in line with the biceps. Exaggerate the opening of the upper back by pressing the chest back towards the feet as much as possible. Hold this position for 5 to 6 breaths.

5. **Utthita Parsvakonasana (Extended Side Angle Pose) –
Insert Extended Angle**

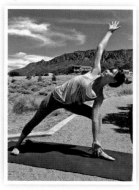

From Down Dog step your left foot forward, bending the knee so the thigh is parallel to the ground and the knee is directly above the ankle. Bring the heel of the back foot to the ground and press through the outer edge. Bring the fingertips your left hand on the ground by your front foot or alternately you can do this pose with your forearm resting on your front thigh. Reach the right arm towards the sky, working to create one line between both arms. Breathe deeply into your lungs as you open the chest by rolling the top ribs back and pressing the bottom ribs forward. Bring your gaze up to the right hand. Stay in this pose for 4 to 5 breaths before stepping back to Down Dog and repeating on the other side.

6. **Lazy Uttanasana (Lazy Standing Forward Bend) –
   Insert Lazy Uttanasana**

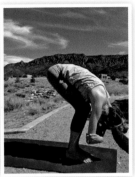

Step forward to the top of your mat. Gently bend the knees and fold forward, lowering your chest onto the thighs. Allow the spine to lengthen by keeping the back of the neck long and heavy. Rest in this position for 6 to 8 breaths.

7. **Padangusthasana (Big Toe Pose),** *alternate variation*

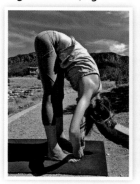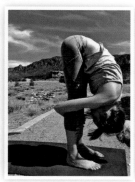

From Lazy Uttanasana, grab onto your big toes with the middle and index fingers, bending the knees if necessary. Use the grip on the toes and the strength of your biceps to fold deeper and open the area in the upper back and between the shoulders.

If the legs are straight after a few breaths in Padangusthasana release the big toes. Reach the hands behind the calves and grab for opposite elbows. Continue folding from the hips. If legs are straight in this position reach the right hand through the legs and grab onto the left shin, left hand reaches for the right shin.

Hold any of the above variations for 5 to 6 breaths before coming to lie on your back in the center of your mat.

8. **Supine Rolls – Supine 1 and 2**

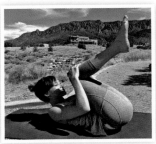

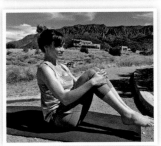

Lying flat on your back, bend your knees and pull them in towards your chest. Begin to rock up and down, massaging the spine. Repeat as many times as you'd like.

9. **Salamba Sarvangasana (Supported Shoulder Stand)**, *variation*

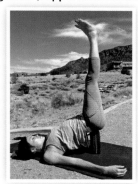

Come to rest on your back with knees bent, feet hip-width apart. Lift the hips off of the ground and place a block right at the base of your spine. There are three levels to a block so choose the height that is appropriate for you (the middle height seems to work best for almost everyone). Place your hands on the block to help hold it in place as you start to lift your feet off of the ground and straighten the legs in the air. You can continue to hold onto your block if you feel more secure, otherwise relax the arms at your sides. Rest in this pose for 1 to 2 minutes.

10. **Setu Bandha Sarvangasana (Supported Bridge Pose),** *variation*

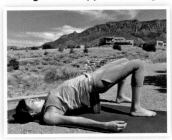

Keeping the block under your low back, lower your feet back to the ground. Plant the soles of the feet firmly into the ground and rest in this supported variation for 1 to 2 minutes. This is a great stress-reliever as well as a great way to reduce pain and tension in the low back.

11. **Savasana (Corpse Pose),** *variation*

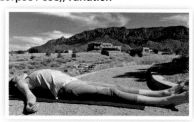

Move your block from your lower back to the space just between your shoulder blades. Lie down with feet extending straight out in front of you, arms at your sides palms up. The back of the head should comfortably touch the ground. If it doesn't, adjust the height of the block.

This variation of Corpse Pose is helpful for opening the chest and improving posture as well as reducing tension in the upper back.

Close your eyes and rest, staying completely still, for as long as you can. Namaste!

OVERTIME
Your Top 10 At Work Yoga Questions Answered

1. **What are the most effective stretches for preventing and relieving carpal tunnel syndrome?**

   Whether you type all day or are just another casualty of smart phone dependence, carpal tunnel syndrome is a serious threat – and it's hitting people younger than ever before. One of the best ways to prevent carpal tunnel and avoid the pain and surgeries that go with it is to keep the joints in the wrists, hands, and fingers healthy with frequent stretching.

Here are five stretches everyone (yes, that includes you) should be doing on a regular basis:

- Finger Stretches

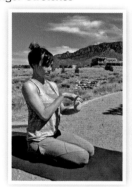 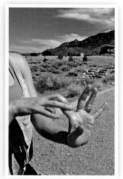

- Reverse Wrist Stretch

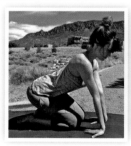 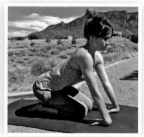

- Eagle Extension

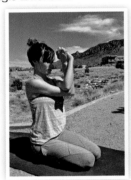 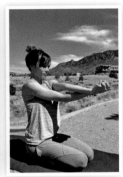

- Knee To Forearm

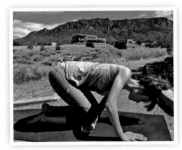

- Gorilla or Kneeling Gorilla

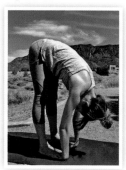

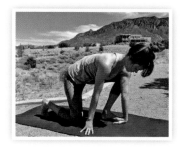

2. **I have no choice but to sit at a desk all day – what should I do?**

If you find yourself stuck at a desk the majority of your day with little to no hope for escape, don't fret! There are still some things you can do to make your time at the office less uncomfortable and less detrimental to your health.

First of all, consider how you sit and what you sit in. Good posture is crucial for good health, which means sit up tall, feet flat on the ground, and shoulders back and away from your ears. Practicing yoga regularly is very helpful for improving posture; so don't forget your pre- and post-work yoga sessions!

And if you are unfortunately stuck sitting all day, you at least have control of what you sit in (or on!) There are lots of office chairs out there that claim to offer amazing support for the low back and supposedly are helpful for maintaining good posture, but keep in mind that these state-of-the-art office chairs come with a hefty price tag. It's also good to remember that while some fancy-pants chairs might make us feel more comfortable during the day, they can actually be causing more damage because they don't give us the feedback we need to know when to correct posture and when to stand up and take a break.

Personally I find that the best option for many people who sit at desks all day is the exercise ball. It's fun, it's bouncy, and it makes you sit up straight. As a bonus, sitting on an exercise ball while you work helps to strengthen your core – who wouldn't want that?

3. **I've heard about companies offering yoga classes during lunch or after work, how do I convince my boss?**

Corporate yoga is gaining popularity globally. More and more companies are offering yoga sessions at no cost to their employees, oftentimes right on site, because not only is it an added perk that keeps their workers happy, but it is also proven to increase productivity as well.

If your work site does not offer yoga classes, a brief conversation with your boss to simply show your interest (and hopefully the interest of others you work with) might be all that it takes. Bosses and companies are always looking for ways to create community among their employees and many are now offering incentives for people who are healthy. What more of an argument do you need when a 30-minute yoga session 3-times a week can be the simple solution to healthy and happy workers?

Unfortunately, not all companies or bosses, even if they understand the benefits of yoga at work and want to offer sessions, can use corporate money to pay for yoga classes. If this is your case, there are still ways to make yoga happen at work you just have to take matters into your own hands. For example, if you can get together with a few of your co-workers, you can contact a local yoga studio and ask about hiring a yoga instructor to come to your place of work during a lunch break or right after work. If a yoga instructor charged $75 per hour for a private session and you could gather a group of 10, then you would each pay less than 8 bucks a session – cheaper than going to a studio and more convenient too!

4. **Not only does my body ache at my desk, but I am stressed out too! What are the best ways to alleviate stress while working?**

Even if you have your dream job, chances are that you will get stressed at work at least once at some point during the week. When stepping away from your desk isn't an option or yoga stretches just don't seem to be cutting it (or you are in the middle of a meeting and whipping your arms into Eagle pose just might seem a bit too weird), utilizing a simple breathing technique is your next best solution.

By simply becoming conscious of how you are breathing (Is it rapid, shallow, are you breathing?) you can begin to change the stressed state you are in. The breath, body, and mind are all intricately connected, which is why breathing techniques are so effective for relaxing body and mind.

Try this simple breath retention technique for an instant calm:

- Begin by taking three deep breaths, breathing in through the nose and deep into the belly and then exhaling completely out through the mouth.
- Then inhale for 2 counts and hold the breath for 2 counts. Repeat this count of inhalation and holding 2 more times (a total of 3) without any exhalation.
- After your third round of retention exhale fully through the mouth.
- Repeat this cycle 5 to 8 times or until your mind and body start to relax, the stress disappears, and clarity returns.

5. **Do I have to bring a yoga mat and change to do yoga at work?**

Of course not! The At-Work session offered in this book is designed to be done at your desk – all you need is a chair. If, however, your work outfit is comprised of a skirt or a dress, you might consider waiting until you lie down with your feet on your chair until you are home!

It's also important to remember that yoga is much more than just stretching. While this book focuses on the physical stretches that often accompany yoga, keep in mind that yoga is learning how to stay present, how to use the breath to keep a calm and positive state of mind, and how to adapt to the changing environment that constantly surrounds us.

6. **Will people think I'm weird if I start doing yoga at my desk?**

I'm not going to lie to you – it's a possibility. But chances are that if anyone does see you practicing a bit of yoga or stretching at work, they will be more curious than anything. From personal experience (and by personal I mean my former boss walking into my classroom, heels in the air, legs up the chair, head under the desk), be prepared to explain what you are doing – not to defend your yoga but because most people will end up wanting you to teach them a stretch or two!

If you do ever receive grief from an at-work yoga session, remember this: you are the healthy one, taking care of your body, and placing importance more on how you feel rather than how you look.

Doing yoga is cool – own it!

7. How often should I take a break and stretch or do some yoga?

A recent article published on Forbes.com highlights a study, known as Organizations in Motion, performed by a group of 750 individuals at New Balance's corporate offices in Boston. The study, which required individuals to get up or stretch every thirty minutes during the work day revealed that in doing this not only were they happier and more comfortable at their desk, but that their engagement and concentration increased throughout the day.

Incorporating regular intervals of exercise or movement into your workday is easier than you might think. Experts say that just doing a couple stretches, standing up and walking to refill a water bottle, or taking a quick break to walk up a flight of stairs and back down again can make a huge difference in your overall health and well being.

8. Why does sitting all day make me so tired?

Lack of movement is your body's way to communicate to your brain that it is time to sleep, which is why long days at the desk leave you feeling more tired than if you were running around all day. Add staring at a screen, which leads to less blinking and tired, dry eyes, to the sedentary jobs the majority of us have, and you have yourself the perfect cocktail of sleepiness.

The solution?

MOVE!
STRETCH!
TRY SOMETHING NEW!
ACT LIKE A KID AGAIN!

1. **Instead of sitting all day I stand all day. Are there any special yoga poses that can help me?**

All this talk about the dangers of too much sitting might lead one to believe that standing is the obvious solution, but this isn't always the case. Bad posture, improper shoes, hard surfaces, can all make standing just as uncomfortable and detrimental as sitting.

If your job requires you to be on your feet for hours at a time, there are a few special yoga poses that will help you stay comfortable and keep your body healthy.

- Tadasana

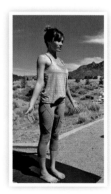

Place a block between your thighs. Press your feet firmly into the ground and evenly distribute your weight through all four corners. Lift the kneecaps to engage the upper legs, but don't lock the knees. Squeeze your thighs against the block and then roll your upper inner thighs back. Imagine your tailbone lengthening towards your heels as you lift your front hip points up.

This pose helps to develop correct posture and prevents you from loading into your low back as you start to fatigue from long bouts of standing.

- Vrksasana

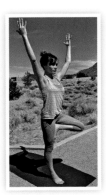

Lift one foot off of the ground, bringing the sole of your foot to the calf, the upper thigh, or the hip crease of the other leg. Your standing leg should be strong and not bending. Gently press your hips forward while you simultaneously press the knee of the lifted leg back. Work on lengthening the spine and the sides of the body. Bring your hands to heart center or raise them over your head, palms facing each other.

In order to balance, keep your eyes focused on one point in front of you. Repeat on the other side.

- Bound Extended Side Angle

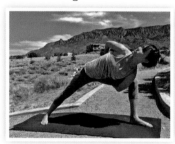

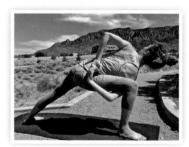

Step your left foot forward, bending the knee so the thigh is parallel to the ground and the knee is directly above the ankle. Bring the heel of the back foot to the ground and press through the outer edge. Bring the fingertips of your left hand on the ground by your front foot. Reach the right arm towards the sky, working to create one line between both arms. Rotate the palm of the right hand behind you and reach back, bending the elbow. Take the left hand off of the ground and reach under your front thigh, clasping the fingers of the right hand. Squeeze the hands together to exaggerate the opening of your chest.

Breathe deeply into your lungs as you open the chest by rolling the top ribs back and pressing the bottom ribs forward. Stay in this pose for 4 to 5 breaths before repeating on the other side.

- Dhanurasana

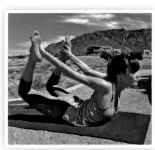

Lying on your stomach, begin to bend the knees, lowering your feet towards your heels. Reach back for your feet, grabbing onto the insides of your ankles, thumbs up. It's very important to keep the knees and ankles in line with your hips as you do this pose, so focus on pulling everything in, arms and legs, towards the center body.

As you inhale, kick the feet back into your hands, lifting the chest off of the ground as you do so. If possible, begin to lift the thighs off of the ground as well, getting a small rocking motion in your hips. Continue to kick up and back higher as you lift the chest and look up. While performing this pose you are increasing flexibility of the total spine, shoulders, and hips, which are all incredibly important for improving posture while both standing and sitting.

- Viparita Karani

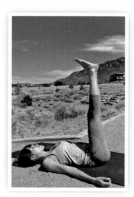

Sidle up as close as you can to a wall so that your entire right side body is touching. Keeping the hips against the wall, swing your legs up and lie down, making a 90-degree angle with your body. Rest, relax, and stay here as long as you can (10 minutes or longer would be ideal) – the benefits are immense for reenergizing the legs, decreasing swelling in the feet and ankles, as well as boosting the immune system and overall mental and physical health!

*Note: This picture demonstrates the posture without a wall, but for full benefits the wall is necessary because it allows you to completely relax without expending energy to keep your feet up in the air.

2. **Work gives me a headache! Can yoga help?**

Yes. In fact, there are yoga postures that are specifically designed to relieve headaches. And as someone who loathes taking pain medication, I use yoga as my primary tool for managing pain – headaches (and childbirth!) included.

Here are the easiest headache-relieving poses that can be done anywhere, anytime, no yoga mat or stretchy pants needed!

- Balasana

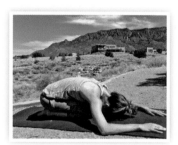

- Balasana with Chair

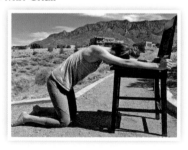

- Neck Stretch – Insert Neck Stretch

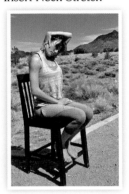

- Relaxed Dolphin – Insert Dolphin

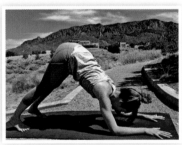

- Savasana with Eye Bag – Insert Bag Savasana

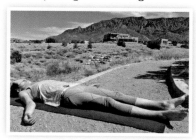

Want To Read More By Julie Schoen?
Check Out Her Amazon Author Page visit:

www.amazon.com/author/julieschoen

Love Yoga?
Check Out The Rest of The Just Do Yoga Series!

GOOD DAY YOGA
GOOD NIGHT YOGA
HAPPY BACK YOGA
FLAT TUMMY YOGA
STRESS LESS YOGA
SUPER IMMUNITY YOGA

Yoginiology.com is the newest lifestyle blog dedicated to writing about the love of yoga, the wonders of the world, and the super powers of women – check it out!

Printed in Great Britain
by Amazon